Kelly Anderson

I0251813

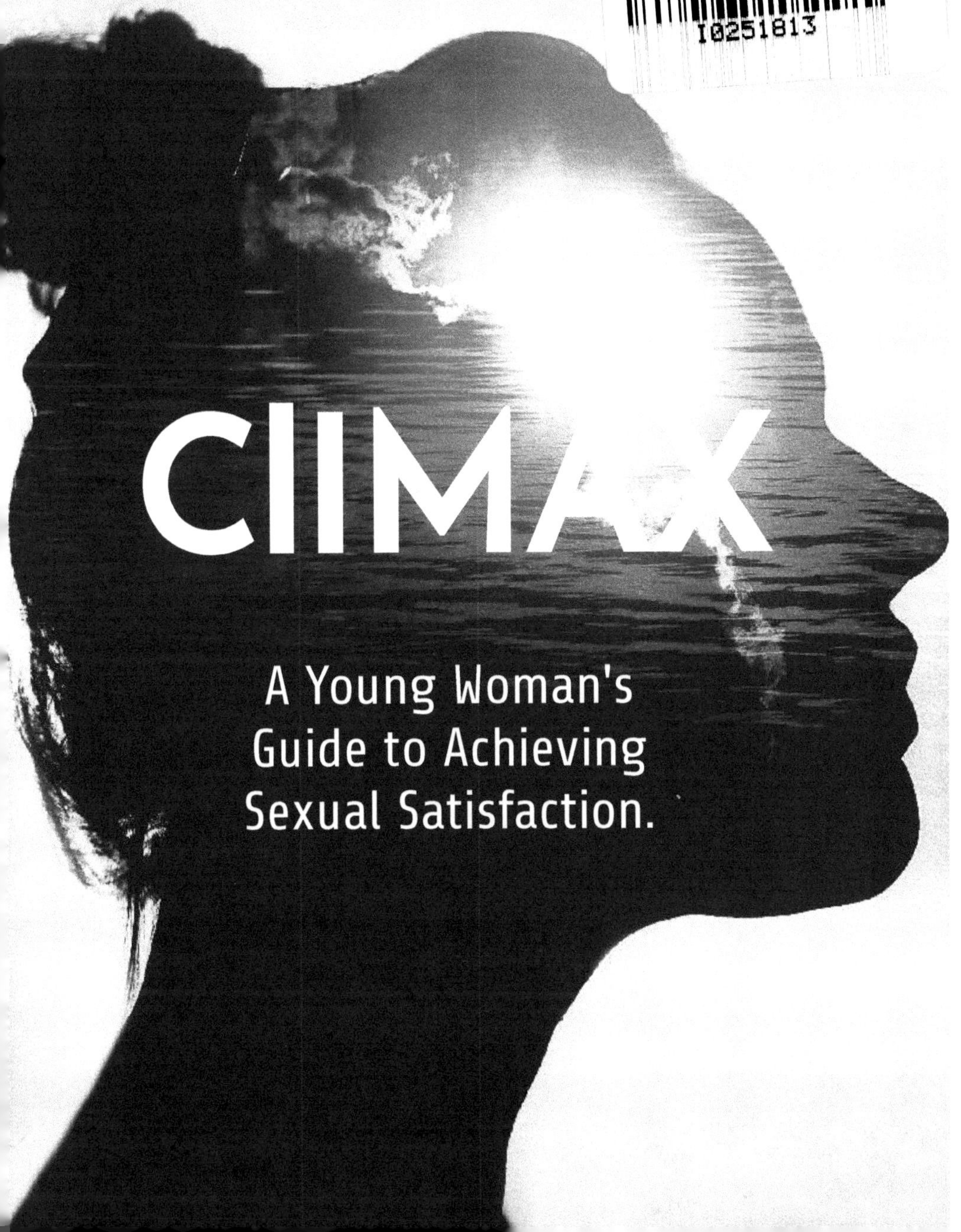

CLIMAX

A Young Woman's Guide to Achieving Sexual Satisfaction.

Table Of Contents

Introduction:

About the author

As the author of Climax: A Young Woman's Guide to Achieving Sexual Satisfaction, I am passionate about empowering women to explore and embrace their sexuality. My name is Kelly, and I have spent years researching and studying the intricacies of female pleasure and sexual health.

Growing up, I was raised in a conservative household where sex was a taboo topic. I was taught to view my sexuality as something shameful and to suppress my desires. However, as I entered adulthood, I realized that this mindset was limiting and harmful. I began to educate myself and explore my sexuality, which led to a newfound sense of confidence and empowerment.

My journey has not been easy, and I have faced many challenges along the way. However, I am determined to share my knowledge and experiences with other young women who may be struggling with similar issues. My goal is to provide them with the tools and information they need to achieve sexual satisfaction and fulfillment.

In addition to being a writer, I am also a certified sex educator and counselor. I have worked with individuals and couples of all ages and backgrounds, helping them to navigate their sexual desires and overcome any obstacles they may be facing.

I believe that sexual health and self-improvement go hand in hand. When we have a healthy and fulfilling sex life, we feel more confident and empowered in all aspects of our lives. It is my hope that this book will inspire young women to embrace their sexuality and take control of their pleasure and satisfaction.

Thank you for taking the time to read my book, and I hope that it will be a valuable resource for you on your own journey towards sexual fulfillment.

Purpose of the book

The purpose of this book, Climax: A Young Woman's Guide to Achieving Sexual Satisfaction, is to empower young adult females to take control of their sexual experiences and achieve maximum pleasure and satisfaction.

As young women, we are often bombarded with messages about sex that are confusing, conflicting, and often negative. We are told that our bodies are objects to be desired, but also that we should be ashamed of our desires. We are taught that sex is something that men do to women, rather than an experience that we can actively participate in and enjoy.

This book seeks to challenge these harmful messages and provide young women with the tools and knowledge they need to have fulfilling and satisfying sexual experiences. It starts by exploring the biology of sex, including the anatomy of the female body and how it responds to stimulation. It then moves on to discuss the emotional and psychological aspects of sex, including how to communicate your desires and boundaries with your partner.

Throughout the book, readers will find practical tips and exercises designed to help them explore their bodies and their desires. They will learn how to prioritize their own pleasure, rather than feeling like they have to cater to their partner's needs. They will also learn how to overcome common obstacles to sexual satisfaction, such as performance anxiety and body image issues.

Ultimately, the goal of this book is to help young women feel confident, empowered, and in control of their sexual experiences. By providing them with the knowledge and tools they need to achieve sexual satisfaction, we hope to help them build healthy and fulfilling relationships with themselves and others.

What is sexual satisfaction?

Sexual satisfaction is a highly subjective experience, and it can mean different things to different people. At its core, sexual satisfaction refers to a feeling of pleasure and fulfillment that arises from sexual activity. It is an important aspect of physical and emotional well-being, and it can enhance our relationships with ourselves and others.

For many young adult females, sexual satisfaction can be elusive. Between societal pressures, relationship dynamics, and personal insecurities, it can be challenging to achieve a sense of sexual fulfillment. However, it is important to remember that sexual satisfaction is not a one-size-fits-all experience. What works for one person may not work for another, and it's perfectly normal to have different preferences and desires.

One key aspect of sexual satisfaction is communication. Being able to communicate your needs and desires with your partner is essential for a fulfilling sexual experience. Whether it's discussing your boundaries, exploring new fantasies, or simply expressing your pleasure, open communication can help you and your partner better understand and fulfill each other's needs.

Another important factor in sexual satisfaction is self-exploration. Taking the time to explore your own body and understand what brings you pleasure can help you communicate your needs to your partner and enhance your overall sexual experience. This can involve solo exploration, such as masturbation, or exploring with a partner in a safe and consensual manner.

Ultimately, sexual satisfaction is about finding what works for you and your partner, and being open to exploring new experiences and desires. This may involve trying new positions, incorporating sex toys or other props, or simply taking the time to connect emotionally with your partner. By prioritizing communication, self-exploration, and openness, you can achieve a sense of sexual satisfaction that enhances your overall well-being and relationships.

Chapter 1: Understanding Your Body

Anatomy of female genitalia

Understanding your menstrual cycle

Understanding your menstrual cycle is crucial for young adult females who are seeking to achieve sexual satisfaction. Menstruation is a natural process that occurs in a woman's body every month. The menstrual cycle is the series of changes that happen in a woman's body to prepare for pregnancy. It is regulated by hormones and can vary from woman to woman.

The menstrual cycle is divided into four phases - the follicular phase, ovulation phase, luteal phase, and menstruation. The follicular phase starts on the first day of your period and lasts for about 14 days. During this phase, the follicles in the ovaries start to mature, and the lining of the uterus thickens, preparing for implantation.

Ovulation is the next phase, which occurs around day 14 of the menstrual cycle. This is when the matured egg is released from the ovary and travels through the fallopian tube, awaiting fertilization. This is the time when you are most fertile, and it is important to use contraception if you are not planning to conceive.

The luteal phase is the third phase and lasts for around 14 days. If the egg was not fertilized during ovulation, the body prepares to shed the lining of the uterus, leading to menstruation.

Menstruation is the fourth phase and lasts for about 3-7 days. This is when the uterus sheds its lining, and you experience bleeding. It is normal to experience cramps, bloating, and mood swings during this time.

It is essential to understand your menstrual cycle as it can affect your sexual health and satisfaction. For instance, during ovulation, you may experience increased libido and arousal, making it an ideal time for sexual activity. On the other hand, some women may experience discomfort or pain during menstruation, which can affect their sexual desire.

In conclusion, understanding your menstrual cycle is key to achieving sexual satisfaction. It helps you plan your sexual activities, understand your body, and identify any irregularities in your cycle. If you experience any abnormal symptoms or have concerns about your menstrual cycle, it is important to consult a healthcare professional.

The importance of self-exploration

The importance of self-exploration cannot be overstated when it comes to achieving sexual satisfaction. As a young adult female, it is essential to take the time to explore your body, your desires, and your boundaries before engaging in sexual activity with a partner.

Self-exploration can involve a variety of activities, including masturbation, journaling, and meditation. Masturbation is an excellent way to get to know your body and what feels good to you. It can help you learn about your erogenous zones and what type of touch you enjoy. Journaling can be used to reflect on your experiences and emotions, helping you identify any negative thoughts or beliefs that may be holding you back from experiencing sexual pleasure. Meditation can help you become more aware of your body and your sensations, allowing you to be more present during sexual activity.

Self-exploration can also involve exploring your fantasies and desires. It is important to understand what turns you on and what you are comfortable with. This can help you communicate your needs and desires to your partner, leading to a more fulfilling sexual experience for both of you.

Taking the time to explore yourself can also help you build self-confidence and self-esteem. When you know what you want and what feels good to you, you are more likely to feel comfortable expressing your needs and desires to your partner. This can lead to a more positive sexual experience and a stronger, healthier relationship.

In conclusion, self-exploration is a crucial aspect of achieving sexual satisfaction. By taking the time to explore your body, desires, and boundaries, you can build self-confidence, communicate your needs and desires to your partner, and ultimately have a more fulfilling sexual experience. So, take the time to explore yourself and embrace your sexuality – you deserve it!

Chapter 2: Overcoming Shame and Guilt

Understanding societal expectations around female sexuality

Understanding Societal Expectations Around Female Sexuality

As a young woman, you may have already encountered societal expectations surrounding your sexuality. From the media to your family and friends, everyone seems to have an opinion on what you should and shouldn't do in the bedroom. But how do these expectations impact you and your sexual experiences? And how can you navigate them to achieve sexual satisfaction on your own terms?

First, it's important to recognize that many of these expectations are rooted in outdated and harmful beliefs about gender and sexuality. For example, women are often expected to be passive and submissive in sexual situations, while men are expected to be aggressive and dominant. This can lead to a power imbalance that can be uncomfortable or even dangerous for women.

Additionally, there is often a double standard when it comes to sexual behavior. Men are often praised for being sexually active, while women are shamed or called derogatory names for the same behavior. This can lead to feelings of guilt or shame for women who want to explore their sexuality.

It's important to remember that you have the right to make your own choices about your body and your sexuality. You don't have to conform to anyone else's expectations or ideals. You are the only one who knows what feels good and right for you.

One way to navigate societal expectations around female sexuality is to educate yourself about healthy and consensual sexual practices. This can include learning about communication, consent, and boundaries. It's also important to understand that sexual pleasure is not just about penetration or orgasm. There are many ways to experience pleasure and intimacy, and it's up to you to explore what feels best for you.

Finally, it's important to surround yourself with supportive and sex-positive people. This can include friends, partners, or mentors who respect your choices and encourage you to explore your sexuality in a safe and healthy way.

In conclusion, understanding societal expectations around female sexuality is an important part of achieving sexual satisfaction as a young woman. By educating yourself, setting boundaries, and surrounding yourself with supportive people, you can navigate these expectations and explore your sexuality on your own terms.

Letting go of shame and guilt

If you are a young adult female who is struggling to achieve sexual satisfaction, you may be experiencing feelings of shame and guilt. Whether it's due to societal pressure, past experiences, or negative self-talk, shame and guilt can create barriers to sexual pleasure and prevent you from enjoying a healthy and fulfilling sex life.

It's important to understand that shame and guilt are not helpful emotions when it comes to sex. They can make you feel embarrassed, unworthy, and anxious, and they can lead to a cycle of negative thoughts and behaviors. The good news is that you can learn to let go of shame and guilt and embrace your sexuality with confidence and joy.

One way to start letting go of shame and guilt is to examine the sources of these emotions. Are they coming from within yourself or from external sources? Are they based on unrealistic expectations or outdated beliefs about sex? Once you have a better understanding of where your shame and guilt are coming from, you can work on challenging and changing those beliefs.

Another helpful strategy is to practice self-compassion. Instead of beating yourself up for not being "perfect" in bed, remind yourself that everyone has different levels of experience and that it's okay to make mistakes. Treat yourself with kindness and understanding, just as you would a friend who is going through a tough time.

Finally, it's important to communicate with your partner(s) about your needs and desires. Talking openly and honestly about sex can help to break down barriers and reduce feelings of shame and guilt. Remember that sexual pleasure is a shared experience and that your partner(s) want you to feel good and enjoy yourself.

Letting go of shame and guilt can be a process, but it's an important step towards achieving sexual satisfaction and living a more fulfilling life. Embrace your sexuality with confidence and joy, and don't let shame and guilt hold you back from experiencing all the pleasure and happiness that sex can bring.

Embracing your sexuality

Embracing Your Sexuality

As a young woman, it can be difficult to fully embrace your sexuality. Society often tells us that we should be ashamed of our desires and that sex is something that should only be talked about in hushed tones. However, it's time to throw those outdated beliefs out the window and start embracing your sexuality.

Sexuality is a natural and healthy expression of who we are as human beings. It's nothing to be ashamed of or embarrassed about. In fact, embracing your sexuality can lead to increased self-confidence, better relationships, and a more fulfilling sex life.

One way to start embracing your sexuality is to explore your body and learn what feels good. Masturbation is a completely normal and healthy way to do this. It allows you to discover what types of touch and stimulation you enjoy, which can then be communicated to your partner during sexual encounters.

It's also important to communicate your desires and boundaries with your partner. Don't be afraid to speak up if something doesn't feel good or if you want to try something new. Good communication is key to a healthy and satisfying sex life.

Another way to embrace your sexuality is to let go of any shame or guilt you may feel about it. Remember that sex is a natural and normal part of life. You have the right to enjoy it without feeling ashamed or judged.

Finally, remember that your sexuality is just one aspect of who you are. It doesn't define you as a person. Embracing your sexuality can lead to increased self-confidence and a better understanding of yourself, but it's important to remember that you are more than just your sexuality.

In conclusion, embracing your sexuality is an important part of becoming a confident and fulfilled young woman. It allows you to explore your desires, communicate with your partner, and let go of any shame or guilt you may feel. Remember to always prioritize your own needs and desires, and never be afraid to speak up for yourself. By doing so, you'll be well on your way to achieving sexual satisfaction and living your best life.

Chapter 3: Communication and Consent

The importance of communication in sexual relationships

Sexual relationships are an important part of our lives, and communication is crucial to achieving sexual satisfaction. It is important to understand that communication is not just about talking, but also about listening and understanding your partner's needs.

When it comes to sex, many young women feel uncomfortable talking about their desires and needs. This can lead to unsatisfying sexual experiences and even resentment towards their partner. In order to avoid this, it is essential to communicate openly and honestly with your partner.

One of the first steps in effective communication is to establish trust. It is important to create a safe space where both partners feel comfortable sharing their desires. This can be achieved by setting boundaries, showing respect, and being open-minded.

Another important aspect of communication in sexual relationships is the ability to listen. It is important to listen to your partner's needs and desires without judgment or criticism. This will help to build trust and allow for a deeper level of intimacy.

It is also important to understand that communication is an ongoing process. As your relationship evolves and changes, so too will your sexual desires and needs. It is important to check in with your partner regularly and discuss any changes or concerns.

In addition to improving sexual satisfaction, effective communication can also strengthen your overall relationship. By being open and honest with your partner, you can build a deeper level of trust and intimacy. This will help to create a more satisfying and fulfilling relationship both inside and outside of the bedroom.

In conclusion, communication is an essential part of any healthy sexual relationship. By establishing trust, listening to your partner's needs, and maintaining ongoing communication, you can achieve a deeper level of intimacy and sexual satisfaction. So don't be afraid to speak up and communicate your desires – it might just lead to the best sex of your life!

Understanding and giving consent

Understanding and giving consent

Consent is crucial in any sexual encounter. It is the foundation of a healthy sexual relationship. Understanding what consent means and how to give it is essential for young women to achieve sexual satisfaction. Consent means that both parties involved in a sexual encounter are willing participants and have given their explicit permission to engage in sexual activities. Consent can only be given when someone is sober, conscious, and fully aware of the situation.

It is essential to understand that consent is not just about saying yes. It is about actively and enthusiastically engaging in the sexual activity. Consent can be withdrawn at any time, and it is the responsibility of both parties to respect each other's boundaries. Always communicate with your partner and ask for their consent before engaging in any sexual activity. It is also important to listen to your partner's verbal and non-verbal cues. If they seem uncomfortable or hesitant, stop immediately and check-in with them.

Giving consent is just as important as understanding it. You should never feel pressured or obliged to engage in sexual activities. Always trust your gut instinct and only engage in sexual activities if you feel comfortable and willing to do so. If you are unsure, it is okay to say no. Your partner should always respect your decision and never pressure you to do anything you are not comfortable with.

Remember, consent is an ongoing process. Just because you have given consent in the past does not mean you have to continue to do so. You have the right to change your mind at any time. Similarly, just because someone has given you consent in the past does not mean you have their consent for future sexual encounters. Always check-in with your partner and ask for their consent before engaging in any sexual activity.

In conclusion, understanding and giving consent is crucial for young women to achieve sexual satisfaction. It is the foundation of a healthy sexual relationship and should never be taken lightly. Always communicate with your partner, listen to their cues, and trust your gut instinct. Remember, consent is an ongoing process, and you have the right to change your mind at any time.

Speaking up for your needs and desires

Speaking up for your needs and desires is an essential aspect of achieving sexual satisfaction. As a young adult female, it can be challenging to express your needs and desires, especially in a sexual context. However, it is crucial to understand that communication is the key to a fulfilling sexual experience.

One of the reasons why many women struggle with speaking up for their needs and desires is the fear of being judged or rejected. It is vital to remember that sexual satisfaction is a two-way street, and your partner's pleasure is just as important as yours. Therefore, speak up and let your partner know what you want and need to achieve sexual satisfaction.

Another reason why young women struggle with expressing their desires is the lack of knowledge about their bodies and what they want. Therefore, it is essential to explore your body and understand what feels good and what does not. Masturbation is an excellent way to explore your body and understand what turns you on. Once you understand what you want, it becomes easier to communicate your desires to your partner.

It is also crucial to understand that sexual desires and needs are not constant and can change over time. Therefore, it is essential to communicate with your partner and check in with yourself regularly to ensure that your needs and desires are being met.

In conclusion, speaking up for your needs and desires is an essential aspect of achieving sexual satisfaction. It may be challenging at first, but with practice, it becomes easier. Remember to communicate with your partner, explore your body, and check in with yourself regularly. By doing so, you can ensure that your sexual experiences are fulfilling and satisfying.

Chapter 4: Masturbation and Orgasm

What is masturbation?

Masturbation is a natural and healthy form of sexual expression that involves self-stimulation for sexual pleasure or orgasm. It is a common and normal activity that people of all genders and sexual orientations engage in throughout their lives. Despite the stigma and taboo surrounding masturbation, it is a crucial aspect of sexual health and well-being.

Masturbation allows individuals to explore their bodies, understand their sexual preferences, and learn how to achieve orgasm. It is a safe and private way to experience sexual pleasure without the risks of sexually transmitted infections or unwanted pregnancies. Masturbation also helps relieve sexual tension and stress, and can improve sleep and mood.

There are many different ways to masturbate, and what feels pleasurable and satisfying can vary from person to person. Some individuals use their hands, while others may use sex toys or other objects. It is important to use a lubricant to prevent discomfort or injury, and to clean any toys or objects before and after use.

Despite the benefits of masturbation, many people feel shame or guilt about engaging in this activity. This can be due to societal and cultural attitudes that label masturbation as sinful, dirty, or shameful. It is important to challenge these negative beliefs and understand that masturbation is a natural and healthy part of human sexuality.

In conclusion, masturbation is a valuable and important aspect of sexual health and well-being. It is a normal and common activity that allows individuals to explore their bodies, understand their sexual preferences, and experience sexual pleasure. By embracing and celebrating masturbation, young adult females can cultivate a positive and healthy relationship with their own sexuality.

How to masturbate

Achieving orgasm through masturbation

Masturbation is one of the most pleasurable activities that all young women should explore. It is a natural and safe way to explore one's sexuality, learn about one's body, and achieve orgasm. As a young woman, you should understand that masturbation is not something to be ashamed of. It is a natural part of human sexuality, and it is essential to embrace it.

One of the main benefits of masturbation is that it helps you to achieve orgasm. Orgasm is the ultimate sexual experience that involves the release of sexual tension and a feeling of intense pleasure. Achieving orgasm through masturbation is a great way to learn about your body and what turns you on. It also helps you to build your confidence and become more comfortable with your sexuality.

To achieve orgasm through masturbation, you need to create the right environment. Find a quiet and private space where you can relax and feel comfortable. You can use a vibrator or your hands to stimulate your clitoris, which is the most sensitive part of your body. Experiment with different techniques and find what works best for you. Some women prefer to use a circular motion, while others prefer a back and forth motion. It is essential to take your time and not rush the process.

It is also important to understand that achieving orgasm through masturbation may take time. It is not something that happens instantly, and you may need to practice several times before you can achieve it. Don't get discouraged if you don't achieve orgasm right away. It takes time and practice to learn how to orgasm through masturbation.

In conclusion, achieving orgasm through masturbation is a natural and safe way to explore your sexuality and learn about your body. It is important to embrace your sexuality and not be ashamed of it. Take your time, experiment with different techniques, and enjoy the process. Remember, self-love is an essential part of sexual satisfaction.

Chapter 5: Exploring Different Sexual Practices

Different types of sexual practices

Sexual satisfaction is not just about intercourse. There are various types of sexual practices that can help you and your partner experience pleasure and reach climax. Here are some of the different types of sexual practices that you can explore:

1. Oral sex: Also known as fellatio (for men) and cunnilingus (for women), oral sex involves stimulating the genitals through the mouth, lips, and tongue. This can be a great way to experience pleasure and achieve orgasm without penetration.

2. Anal sex: This involves stimulating the anus and rectum with fingers, toys, or a penis. It can be a pleasurable experience for both men and women, but it should be practiced with caution and plenty of lubrication.

3. BDSM: This stands for bondage, domination, submission, and masochism. BDSM involves exploring power dynamics and sexual fantasies through activities such as spanking, role-playing, and using restraints. It can be a consensual and exciting way to spice up your sex life.

4. Mutual masturbation: This involves stimulating yourself while your partner watches or stimulates themselves at the same time. It can be a great way to build intimacy and learn more about your partner's desires.

5. Kissing and touching: Sometimes, simple acts like kissing, touching, and caressing can be just as pleasurable as more explicit sexual activities. Don't underestimate the power of a good make-out session!

Remember, it's important to communicate with your partner about what you're comfortable with and to always practice safe sex. By exploring different types of sexual practices, you can discover what brings you the most pleasure and achieve sexual satisfaction in new and exciting ways.

Understanding and exploring your sexual fantasies

Understanding and exploring your sexual fantasies is an essential part of discovering your sexual identity. It allows you to explore your desires, understand what turns you on, and communicate your needs to your partner. Sexual fantasies are a healthy and normal part of human sexuality, and they can be a powerful tool for self-discovery and sexual empowerment.

It is important to note that sexual fantasies are personal and varied. What turns one person on may not be the same for another. However, some common themes include power dynamics, role-playing, and exploring taboo subjects. These fantasies can range from mild to extreme, but it is important to remember that they are only a fantasy and do not necessarily reflect your real-life desires or actions.

Exploring your sexual fantasies can be a fun and exciting way to get to know yourself better. You can start by writing down your fantasies in a journal or sharing them with a trusted partner or friend. It is important to remember that fantasies are not a reflection of reality, and it is okay to have secret desires that you do not want to act on.

It is also important to communicate your desires and boundaries with your partner. Consent is crucial in any sexual encounter, and discussing your fantasies can be a great way to explore your desires in a safe and consensual way.

In conclusion, understanding and exploring your sexual fantasies is an important part of self-discovery and sexual empowerment. It allows you to explore your desires, communicate your needs, and engage in consensual sexual experiences. Remember that your sexual fantasies are personal and varied, and there is no right or wrong way to explore them. Embrace your desires and have fun exploring your sexuality.

Experimenting with different sexual positions

Experimenting with Different Sexual Positions

Sexual satisfaction is about more than just achieving orgasm. It's about exploring your body and your partner's body in new and exciting ways. One way to do this is by experimenting with different sexual positions.

There are countless positions to try, each with its own unique benefits. Some positions may be more comfortable for you and your partner, while others may be more intimate or allow for deeper penetration. The key is to find what works best for you and your partner.

One popular position is missionary, where the woman lies on her back and the man lies on top of her. This position allows for eye contact and intimacy, and can also allow for deeper penetration. Another popular position is doggy style, where the woman is on all fours and the man enters from behind. This position can allow for deeper penetration and can be a turn-on for many couples.

Other positions to try include cowgirl, where the woman is on top and in control, and the spooning position, where both partners lie on their sides and the man enters from behind. The possibilities are endless, and it's important to be open to trying new things.

It's also important to communicate with your partner about what feels good and what doesn't. Don't be afraid to speak up and guide your partner to the right spot. Remember, sex is about pleasure for both partners, and communication is key to achieving that pleasure.

In addition to trying different positions, incorporating sex toys into your sex life can also add excitement and pleasure. Vibrators, dildos, and other toys can be used alone or with a partner to enhance sexual pleasure.

Experimenting with different sexual positions and incorporating sex toys into your sex life can be a fun and exciting way to explore your sexuality and achieve sexual satisfaction. Remember to communicate with your partner, be open to trying new things, and most importantly, have fun!

Chapter 6: Dealing with Sexual Dysfunction

Understanding sexual dysfunction

Sexual dysfunction is a common issue that affects people of all genders and ages. It is a condition where a person experiences difficulty in achieving sexual satisfaction or experiencing pleasure during sexual activity. Sexual dysfunction can be caused by various factors, including physical, psychological, and emotional issues.

Physical factors that can affect sexual function include hormonal imbalances, chronic illnesses, medications, and surgeries. Psychological factors include anxiety, depression, stress, and trauma. Emotional factors such as relationship problems, low self-esteem, and fear of intimacy can also contribute to sexual dysfunction.

Some of the common types of sexual dysfunction include low libido, difficulty achieving orgasm, pain during intercourse, and erectile dysfunction. Low libido is a lack of sexual desire, while difficulty achieving orgasm is the inability to reach orgasm despite sexual stimulation. Pain during intercourse can be caused by a variety of factors, including infections, vaginismus, and endometriosis. Erectile dysfunction is the inability to achieve or maintain an erection during sexual activity.

It is important to note that sexual dysfunction is not a reflection of a person's worth or value. It is a medical condition that can be treated and managed with the help of a healthcare professional. Treatment options for sexual dysfunction vary depending on the underlying cause. For example, if the cause is physical, medication or surgery may be recommended. If the cause is psychological, therapy or counseling may be recommended.

In conclusion, sexual dysfunction is a common issue that affects many people. It is important to seek help if you are experiencing any symptoms of sexual dysfunction. Remember that you are not alone and that there are treatment options available to help you achieve sexual satisfaction and improve your overall sexual health.

Common causes of sexual dysfunction

Sexual dysfunction can be a sensitive and challenging topic, but it's important to know that it's not uncommon and there are ways to address it. Sexual dysfunction refers to any difficulty or issue that prevents an individual from experiencing sexual satisfaction or pleasure. It can affect anyone, regardless of age or gender, but it's particularly prevalent among young adult females. In this subchapter, we'll discuss some of the most common causes of sexual dysfunction.

1. Anxiety and Stress

Anxiety and stress can be significant factors that impact sexual function. When you're feeling anxious or stressed, your body produces cortisol, a hormone that can affect sexual desire and arousal. Additionally, anxiety can cause performance anxiety, making it difficult to relax and enjoy sexual experiences.

2. Hormonal Imbalances

Hormonal imbalances can also cause sexual dysfunction. When your body's hormones are imbalanced, it can affect your libido, arousal, and ability to experience orgasm. Hormonal imbalances can be caused by a variety of factors, including pregnancy, menopause, and certain medications.

3. Medical Conditions

Certain medical conditions can also cause sexual dysfunction. Conditions such as diabetes, heart disease, and multiple sclerosis can all impact sexual function. Additionally, chronic pain or fatigue can make it difficult to engage in sexual activity.

4. Relationship Issues

Relationship issues can also impact sexual function. Communication problems, unresolved conflicts, and lack of intimacy can all contribute to sexual dysfunction. It's essential to address any relationship issues to improve sexual satisfaction.

5. Negative Body Image

Negative body image can also contribute to sexual dysfunction. If you're not comfortable with your body, it can be challenging to feel confident and sexy during sexual experiences. It's important to work on improving your body image to improve sexual satisfaction.

In conclusion, sexual dysfunction is a common issue that can affect young adult females. By understanding some of the common causes, you can take steps to address the issue and improve sexual satisfaction. It's essential to speak with a healthcare provider if you're experiencing sexual dysfunction to identify any underlying medical issues and develop a treatment plan.

Seeking professional help

Sexual satisfaction is a crucial aspect of our lives, as it affects our physical, emotional, and psychological wellbeing. However, achieving sexual satisfaction is not always easy, and it is common to encounter challenges and obstacles along the way. If you are struggling to achieve sexual satisfaction, seeking professional help could be a game-changer.

Professional help can come in many forms, including therapy, coaching, and medical treatment. Seeking help from a qualified professional can help you identify the underlying issues that are preventing you from achieving sexual satisfaction, and they can provide you with the tools and resources you need to overcome these challenges.

Therapy is an excellent option for those who are struggling with psychological or emotional barriers to sexual satisfaction. A therapist can help you work through past trauma, negative self-talk, or relationship issues that may be impacting your ability to enjoy sex and achieve orgasm. They can also teach you mindfulness techniques and coping strategies to help you manage anxiety and stress that may be interfering with your sexual pleasure.

Coaching is another option for those who are looking to improve their sexual skills and enhance their overall sexual experience. Sex coaches can provide you with practical advice and guidance on how to communicate your desires, explore new sexual experiences, and develop a better understanding of your body and sexual needs.

Medical treatment may also be necessary for some individuals who are struggling with physical barriers to sexual satisfaction. For example, a doctor may prescribe medication to treat conditions such as depression, anxiety, or chronic pain, which can all impact sexual function.

In conclusion, seeking professional help is a vital step towards achieving sexual satisfaction. Whether you are struggling with psychological, emotional, or physical barriers to sexual pleasure, there are qualified professionals who can help you overcome these challenges and empower you to enjoy a fulfilling and satisfying sex life.

Chapter 7: Sexual Health and Safety

Understanding STIs and contraception

Understanding STIs and contraception is crucial for young adult females who are sexually active or planning to be. Sexually transmitted infections (STIs) are infections that can be transmitted from one person to another during sexual contact. These infections can be caused by bacteria, viruses, or parasites and can have serious consequences if left untreated.

The most common STIs include chlamydia, gonorrhea, syphilis, and HIV/AIDS. The symptoms of these infections may not be noticeable at first, which is why it is important to get tested regularly if you are sexually active. You can get tested for STIs at your local health clinic or your healthcare provider. Some STIs can be treated with antibiotics, while others are incurable but can be managed with medication.

One of the best ways to protect yourself from STIs is to use contraception during sexual activity. Contraception is any method used to prevent pregnancy or STIs. There are many different types of contraception available, including condoms, birth control pills, intrauterine devices (IUDs), and implants.

Condoms are one of the most effective methods of contraception because they not only prevent pregnancy but also protect against STIs. Birth control pills are another popular method, but they do not protect against STIs. It is important to talk to your healthcare provider to determine which method of contraception is right for you.

Remember that STIs can be passed through oral, vaginal, and anal sex, so it is important to use protection every time you engage in sexual activity. If you are unsure about your partner's sexual history or if you suspect that you may have an STI, it is crucial to get tested and treated as soon as possible.

In conclusion, understanding STIs and contraception is essential for young adult females who are sexually active or planning to be. Protecting yourself from STIs and unintended pregnancies is the first step towards achieving sexual satisfaction and taking control of your sexual health. Don't be afraid to talk to your healthcare provider or seek information from reputable sources to learn more about STIs and contraception.

Taking care of your sexual health

Taking care of your sexual health is an essential part of being a sexually active young adult female. It can help you avoid unwanted pregnancies, sexually transmitted infections (STIs), and ensure that you have a pleasurable and satisfying sexual experience.

One of the first steps to taking care of your sexual health is to educate yourself about sex and STIs. You should know the signs and symptoms of common STIs and how to practice safe sex. This includes using condoms and other forms of contraception, getting regular STI testing, and being open and honest with your sexual partners about your sexual health.

Another important aspect of sexual health is maintaining good hygiene. This means keeping your genitals clean and dry, wearing clean underwear, and avoiding harsh soaps and perfumes that can irritate the sensitive skin in your genital area.

It's also important to prioritize your own pleasure and communication with your partner. Many young women feel pressured to prioritize their partner's pleasure over their own, but this can lead to dissatisfaction and discomfort. It's important to communicate with your partner about your desires and boundaries and prioritize your own pleasure.

If you do experience any discomfort or pain during sex, it's important to seek medical attention. Pain during sex can be a sign of an underlying medical condition, and it's important to get treatment as soon as possible.

Taking care of your sexual health also means taking care of your mental and emotional health. Sex can be an emotionally charged experience, and it's important to prioritize your own mental and emotional well-being. This means communicating with your partner, setting boundaries, and being honest with yourself about your own desires and needs.

In conclusion, taking care of your sexual health is essential for young adult females. It involves educating yourself about sex and STIs, maintaining good hygiene, prioritizing your own pleasure and communication with your partner, seeking medical attention when necessary, and taking care of your mental and emotional health. By taking these steps, you can ensure that you have a pleasurable and satisfying sexual experience while also protecting your overall health and wellbeing.

Staying safe in sexual relationships

and "relationships."

Sexual relationships are a part of many young adults' lives, and it's important to stay safe while exploring your sexuality. Whether you're in a committed relationship or enjoying casual encounters, there are steps you can take to protect yourself and your partner.

First, make sure you're comfortable with your partner and that you trust them. If you're not sure about their intentions or if they're pressuring you, it's okay to say no and walk away. You have the right to make your own choices about your body and your sexual experiences.

Next, always use protection. Condoms are the most effective way to prevent sexually transmitted infections (STIs) and unintended pregnancies. Make sure you have a supply of condoms on hand and feel comfortable talking to your partner about using them.

It's also important to get tested regularly for STIs, especially if you're sexually active with multiple partners. Many STIs can be asymptomatic, meaning you may not even know you have them. Getting tested regularly can help you catch and treat infections early, preventing long-term health complications.

Communication is key in any relationship, but especially when it comes to sexual relationships. Talk to your partner about your boundaries, desires, and concerns. If something doesn't feel right or if you're unsure about a situation, speak up and ask questions. Your partner should respect your boundaries and make sure you feel safe and comfortable at all times.

Lastly, trust your instincts. If something feels off or if you're uncomfortable with a situation, it's okay to say no and walk away. Your safety and well-being should always come first.

In conclusion, staying safe in sexual relationships is crucial for young adults. By trusting your partner, using protection, getting tested regularly, communicating openly, and trusting your instincts, you can enjoy fulfilling and satisfying sexual experiences while also prioritizing your health and safety.

Chapter 8: Conclusion

Recap of key points

Recap of Key Points

Throughout this book, we have covered a lot of ground when it comes to achieving sexual satisfaction. Whether you're in a committed relationship or exploring your sexuality as a single woman, there are a few key points to keep in mind.

First and foremost, communication is key. You and your partner(s) need to be able to talk openly and honestly about your desires, needs, and boundaries. This can be intimidating, but it's vital if you want to have a fulfilling sex life.

Secondly, it's important to remember that pleasure is a two-way street. You deserve to feel good, and so does your partner. Don't be afraid to ask for what you want, and don't be shy about exploring your partner's body and learning what they enjoy.

Another key point is that there is no "right" or "wrong" way to have sex. Everyone's preferences are different, and that's okay. What matters most is that you and your partner(s) are comfortable, safe, and enjoying yourselves.

It's also worth noting that sexual satisfaction is about more than just physical pleasure. Emotional intimacy, trust, and respect are all important components of a healthy sexual relationship. Take the time to build these connections with your partner(s) and prioritize your emotional wellbeing.

Finally, it's important to remember that sexual satisfaction is a journey, not a destination. Your preferences and desires may change over time, and that's okay. Keep an open mind and stay curious about your own sexuality and that of your partner(s).

In conclusion, achieving sexual satisfaction is about more than just technique or physical pleasure. It requires communication, trust, emotional intimacy, and an open mind. By keeping these key points in mind, you can enjoy a fulfilling and satisfying sex life, whether you're single or in a committed relationship.

Embracing your sexuality and achieving sexual satisfaction

Embracing your sexuality and achieving sexual satisfaction is a crucial part of a young woman's life. It is essential to understand your body, desires, and needs to lead a fulfilling sexual life. Unfortunately, society often shames women for their sexuality and labels them as promiscuous or immoral. However, it's time to break free from these societal stereotypes and embrace your sexuality.

To achieve sexual satisfaction, it is vital to understand your body. Take the time to explore your body, understand what turns you on, and what doesn't. Use this knowledge to communicate your needs to your partner. Communication is key when it comes to sexual satisfaction. Don't be afraid to voice your desires and preferences to your partner. It's essential to be comfortable with your partner and trust them to make sex enjoyable for both of you.

It's also important to understand that sexual satisfaction is not just about the physical act of sex. It's about the emotional and mental connection with your partner. Take the time to build a connection with your partner, and the physical aspect of sex will come naturally.

Along with understanding your body, it's important to prioritize your sexual health. Get regular check-ups, use protection, and practice safe sex. It's essential to take care of your sexual health to avoid any complications or diseases that can hinder your sexual satisfaction.

Lastly, don't be afraid to try new things. Experimenting with different positions, toys, and fantasies can enhance your sexual experience and bring excitement to your sex life. Remember, there's no right or wrong way to have sex, as long as it's consensual and enjoyable for both partners.

In conclusion, embracing your sexuality and achieving sexual satisfaction is a journey. It takes time, patience, and communication with your partner. However, it's essential to prioritize your sexual health, understand your body, and not be afraid to try new things. By doing so, you can lead a fulfilling and satisfying sexual life.

Final thoughts and resources.

Final Thoughts and Resources

Congratulations on finishing Climax: A Young Woman's Guide to Achieving Sexual Satisfaction! We hope that you've found the book informative and helpful in your journey towards sexual empowerment and fulfillment.

As we come to the end of this book, we want to leave you with some final thoughts and resources that we believe will be useful as you continue on your path towards sexual satisfaction.

Firstly, we want to remind you that achieving sexual satisfaction is a journey, not a destination. It's important to keep exploring and experimenting with different techniques and approaches to find what works best for you. Don't be afraid to communicate your wants and needs with your partner(s) and to try new things.

We also want to emphasize the importance of consent and communication in sexual relationships. It's crucial to always ask for and respect your partner's boundaries and to have open and honest conversations about your desires and expectations.

In addition to sexual satisfaction, we believe that self-improvement and personal growth are important aspects of a fulfilling life. Take the time to invest in yourself, whether that means pursuing your passions, practicing self-care, or seeking therapy or counseling when needed.

Finally, we want to provide you with some additional resources that we believe may be helpful in your journey towards sexual empowerment and personal growth:

- The Scarleteen website (https://www.scarleteen.com/) provides comprehensive sex education and advice for young people.

- The Clue period tracking app (https://helloclue.com/) can help you track your menstrual cycle and better understand your body's hormonal changes.

- The book Come as You Are by Emily Nagoski is an excellent resource for understanding female sexuality and achieving sexual satisfaction.

- The podcast Sex with Emily (https://sexwithemily.com/podcast/) provides informative and engaging discussions on all aspects of sex and relationships.

We hope that you've found Climax to be a valuable resource in your journey towards sexual satisfaction and personal growth. Remember, you deserve to experience pleasure and fulfillment in your sexual relationships, and we believe in your ability to achieve it. Good luck!

Climax: A Young Woman's Guide to Achieving Sexual Satisfaction.

Best of luck & love in your sexual adventures... until next time! - Kelly :)

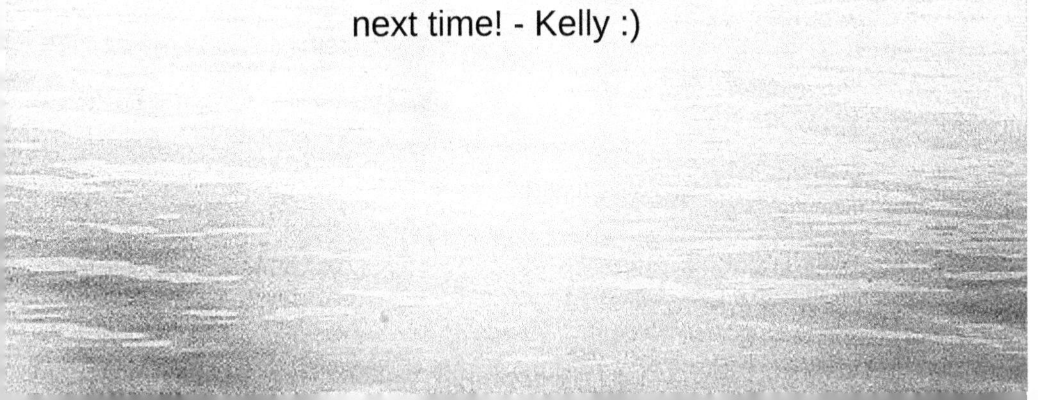

www.ingramcontent.com/pod-product-compliance
Lightning Source LLC
Chambersburg PA
CBHW071727020426
42333CB00017B/2427
* 9 7 8 1 0 8 8 1 9 9 1 7 6 *